DOCTOR BARBARA SIMPLE CURE FOR CANCER

Unlocking natural healing: discover Dr Barbara's revolutionary approach conquering cancer with holistic remedies and transformative lifestyle choices

Edwardo Pedro

Table of Contents

COPYRIGHT © 2023

CHAPTER ONE

Introduction to Dr. Barbara's Approach to Herbal Cancer Treatment

Dr. Barbara's approach to herbal cancer treatment represents a comprehensive and holistic perspective on addressing cancer using natural remedies derived from plants. It combines traditional herbal medicine knowledge with modern scientific research to develop protocols that aim to support the body's innate healing mechanisms while minimizing side effects. This approach acknowledges the complexity of cancer and recognizes the importance of integrating various modalities to achieve optimal outcomes.

At the core of Dr. Barbara's approach is the belief in the synergy of plant compounds and their ability to exert multifaceted effects on cancer cells, the immune system, and overall health. This holistic perspective views cancer as not just a localized disease but as a manifestation of underlying imbalances within the body's systems. By addressing these imbalances through herbal interventions, Dr. Barbara aims to restore harmony and enhance the body's ability to fight cancer naturally.

Understanding Cancer from a Holistic Perspective

To appreciate Dr. Barbara's approach, it's essential to understand cancer from a holistic perspective. Cancer is not merely a result of genetic mutations or abnormal cell growth but a complex interplay of various factors, including genetic predisposition, environmental influences, lifestyle choices, and immune function. Holistic medicine recognizes that these factors are interconnected and that addressing them comprehensively is key to effective cancer treatment and prevention.

From Dr. Barbara's viewpoint, cancer arises when the body's natural defense mechanisms become compromised, allowing abnormal cells to proliferate unchecked. This could result from factors such as chronic inflammation, oxidative stress, immune dysfunction, hormonal imbalances, or toxin exposure. Rather than targeting cancer cells alone, Dr. Barbara's approach seeks to create an internal environment that is inhospitable to cancer growth while supporting the body's ability to identify and eliminate abnormal cells.

The Role of Herbal Medicine in Cancer Treatment

Herbal medicine has been used for centuries to treat various ailments, including cancer. Plants contain a diverse array of bioactive compounds, many of which have demonstrated anticancer properties in laboratory studies and clinical trials. Unlike conventional cancer treatments such as chemotherapy and radiation therapy, which often have significant side effects, herbal remedies are generally well-tolerated and can be tailored to individual needs.

Dr. Barbara's approach involves selecting specific herbs based on their known or potential anticancer properties and formulating them into personalized treatment protocols. These protocols may include a combination of herbs taken orally, applied topically, or administered via other routes such as intravenous infusion or enema. By harnessing the synergistic effects of multiple herbs, Dr. Barbara aims to enhance their overall efficacy while minimizing the risk of resistance or adverse reactions.

Principles of Herbal Cancer Treatment

Dr. Barbara's approach to herbal cancer treatment is guided by several key principles:

1. **Individualized Treatment**: Each patient is unique, and their cancer treatment should reflect their specific needs, preferences, and medical history. Dr. Barbara conducts a thorough assessment of each patient's health status, including their cancer type, stage, genetic profile, and overall constitution, to tailor a personalized treatment plan.

2. **Multimodal Approach**: Cancer is a multifaceted disease, and effective treatment often requires addressing multiple factors simultaneously. Dr. Barbara integrates various modalities such as herbal medicine, nutrition, lifestyle modifications, mind-body practices, and conventional therapies to create a comprehensive treatment strategy.

3. **Supporting the Body's Healing Response**: Rather than directly targeting cancer cells with toxic agents, Dr. Barbara's approach focuses on supporting the body's innate healing mechanisms. This involves strengthening the immune system, reducing inflammation, enhancing detoxification pathways, and promoting overall vitality and resilience.

4. **Emphasis on Prevention and Maintenance**: In addition to treating existing cancer, Dr. Barbara emphasizes the importance of prevention and long-term maintenance. This includes lifestyle modifications, dietary changes, ongoing herbal support, regular monitoring, and proactive management of risk factors to reduce the likelihood of cancer recurrence or progression.

Evidence-Based Herbal Therapies

While traditional herbal medicine provides a rich source of knowledge, Dr. Barbara's approach also incorporates modern scientific research to validate the efficacy and safety of herbal therapies. Numerous studies have investigated the anticancer properties of various herbs and plant compounds, elucidating their mechanisms of action and potential synergies.

For example, herbs such as turmeric (Curcuma longa), green tea (Camellia sinensis), reishi mushroom (Ganoderma lucidum), and astragalus (Astragalus membranaceus) have been extensively studied for their anticancer effects. These herbs contain bioactive compounds such as curcumin, epigallocatechin gallate (EGCG), polysaccharides, and astragalosides, which have demonstrated inhibitory effects on cancer cell growth, metastasis, angiogenesis, and inflammation.

In addition to single herbs, Dr. Barbara often formulates complex herbal blends designed to target multiple pathways involved in cancer development and progression. These formulations may include synergistic combinations of herbs, vitamins, minerals, antioxidants, and other nutrients aimed at enhancing efficacy and minimizing side effects.

Clinical Application and Case Studies

Dr. Barbara's approach to herbal cancer treatment has been applied successfully in clinical practice, yielding positive outcomes for many patients. Case studies provide valuable insights into the practical application of herbal therapies and illustrate their potential effectiveness in real-world settings.

One such case involves a 55-year-old female diagnosed with stage II breast cancer who opted for a holistic treatment approach. In addition to conventional therapies such as surgery and radiation, she received personalized herbal formulations targeting inflammation, immune support, and hormone balance. Over the course of six months, her tumor markers decreased, and imaging studies showed a reduction in tumor size without significant side effects.

Another case involves a 68-year-old male with stage IV prostate cancer who chose to pursue herbal therapy as an adjunct to conventional treatment. He received a combination of herbs known for their anti-inflammatory, antioxidant, and immune-modulating properties, along with dietary and lifestyle recommendations. Despite the advanced stage of his cancer, he experienced improvements in quality of life, symptom management, and overall survival compared to historical outcomes.

Challenges and Considerations

While herbal medicine offers promising potential in cancer treatment, several challenges and considerations must be addressed:

1. **Quality and Standardization**: Ensuring the quality, purity, and consistency of herbal products is essential for optimal therapeutic outcomes. Dr. Barbara sources herbs from

reputable suppliers and prioritizes organic, sustainably harvested, and rigorously tested ingredients to minimize contamination and variability.

2. **Drug-Herb Interactions**: Some herbs may interact with medications commonly used in cancer treatment, potentially altering their efficacy or safety profiles. Dr. Barbara conducts thorough evaluations of patients' medication regimens and adjusts herbal protocols accordingly to minimize the risk of interactions.

3. **Patient Compliance and Education**: Herbal treatment requires active participation and commitment from patients, including adherence to prescribed protocols, lifestyle modifications, and ongoing monitoring. Dr. Barbara emphasizes patient education, empowerment, and support to facilitate informed decision-making and long-term success.

4. **Integration with Conventional Care**: Herbal medicine should complement, rather than replace, conventional cancer treatments such as surgery, chemotherapy, and radiation therapy. Dr. Barbara collaborates closely with oncologists and other healthcare providers to ensure seamless integration of herbal therapies into comprehensive cancer care plans.

In conclusion, Dr. Barbara's approach to herbal cancer treatment offers a holistic, evidence-based, and patient-centered alternative to conventional therapies. By leveraging the therapeutic potential of medicinal plants in synergy with modern scientific understanding, Dr. Barbara aims to empower patients to take an active role in their healing journey while promoting optimal health and well-being.

CHAPTER TWO

Understanding Cancer: Causes, Types, and Conventional Treatments

Cancer, a multifaceted and complex group of diseases, is characterized by the abnormal growth and spread of cells. It remains one of the leading causes of morbidity and mortality worldwide. Understanding the causes, types, and conventional treatments of cancer is crucial for effective prevention, diagnosis, and management.

Causes of Cancer

Cancer is not caused by a single factor but arises from a combination of genetic, environmental, and lifestyle influences. Several key factors contribute to the development of cancer:

1. **Genetic Mutations**: Mutations in specific genes can disrupt normal cell growth and division, leading to uncontrolled proliferation and tumor formation. These mutations can be inherited (germline mutations) or acquired over time due to exposure to carcinogens, radiation, or errors in DNA replication.

2. **Environmental Exposures**: Exposure to carcinogenic substances in the environment, such as tobacco smoke, asbestos, ultraviolet radiation, certain chemicals, and pollutants, can increase the risk of developing cancer. These

substances can damage DNA, promote inflammation, and disrupt cellular processes, predisposing cells to malignant transformation.

3. **Lifestyle Factors**: Certain lifestyle choices, including tobacco use, excessive alcohol consumption, unhealthy diet, physical inactivity, and obesity, contribute to cancer development. These factors can influence cellular metabolism, hormone levels, immune function, and inflammation, creating an environment conducive to cancer growth.

4. **Infectious Agents**: Some cancers are caused by infectious agents such as viruses, bacteria, and parasites. For example, human papillomavirus (HPV) is linked to cervical, anal, and oropharyngeal cancers, while Helicobacter pylori infection is associated with stomach cancer.

5. **Hormonal Imbalances**: Hormonal imbalances, such as elevated levels of estrogen or testosterone, can promote the growth of hormone-sensitive cancers such as breast, prostate, and ovarian cancer. Hormone replacement therapy, oral contraceptives, and certain medical conditions may alter hormone levels and increase cancer risk.

Types of Cancer

Cancer can arise in almost any tissue or organ of the body and is classified based on its tissue of origin, histological characteristics, and molecular features. Some of the most common types of cancer include:

1. **Carcinomas**: These cancers originate from epithelial cells, which line the surfaces and cavities of organs throughout the body. Carcinomas account for the majority of cancer cases and include subtypes such as lung cancer, breast cancer, prostate cancer, colorectal cancer, and skin cancer (melanoma and non-melanoma).

2. **Sarcomas**: Sarcomas arise from connective tissues such as bone, muscle, cartilage, and fat. They are less common than carcinomas but can be highly aggressive. Examples of sarcomas include osteosarcoma (bone cancer), leiomyosarcoma (smooth muscle cancer), and liposarcoma (fat tissue cancer).

3. **Lymphomas**: Lymphomas originate from lymphocytes, a type of white blood cell involved in the immune system. They typically arise in lymphoid tissues such as lymph nodes, spleen, and bone marrow. Hodgkin lymphoma and non-Hodgkin lymphoma are the two main types of lymphoma.

4. **Leukemias**: Leukemias are cancers of the blood and bone marrow, where abnormal white blood cells proliferate uncontrollably and interfere with normal blood cell production. Leukemias are classified based on the type of white blood cell affected, including lymphocytic leukemia

(affecting lymphocytes) and myeloid leukemia (affecting other types of white blood cells).

5. **Central Nervous System (CNS) Tumors**: CNS tumors arise in the brain or spinal cord and can be either benign or malignant. They can cause neurological symptoms and complications depending on their location and size. Examples include gliomas, meningiomas, and medulloblastomas.

Conventional Treatments for Cancer

Conventional treatments for cancer aim to eradicate or control malignant cells while minimizing damage to normal tissues. Several modalities are commonly used alone or in combination, depending on the type and stage of cancer:

1. **Surgery**: Surgical removal of cancerous tissue is often performed if the tumor is localized and can be safely excised. Surgery may be curative for early-stage cancers or used to alleviate symptoms and improve quality of life in advanced cases.

2. **Chemotherapy**: Chemotherapy involves the use of cytotoxic drugs to kill rapidly dividing cancer cells or inhibit their growth. Chemotherapy may be administered orally, intravenously, or topically and is often used in combination with other treatments such as surgery and radiation therapy.

3. **Radiation Therapy**: Radiation therapy uses high-energy beams of radiation to destroy cancer cells or prevent their proliferation. It can be delivered externally (external beam radiation) or internally (brachytherapy) and is commonly used as a primary treatment or adjuvant therapy following surgery.

4. **Immunotherapy**: Immunotherapy harnesses the body's immune system to recognize and attack cancer cells. It includes various approaches such as immune checkpoint inhibitors, monoclonal antibodies, adoptive cell therapy, and cancer vaccines. Immunotherapy has revolutionized cancer treatment and shown promising results in certain cancers.

5. **Targeted Therapy**: Targeted therapy targets specific molecular pathways or genetic alterations driving cancer growth and progression. It includes drugs that inhibit oncogenic proteins, signaling pathways, or angiogenesis (formation of new blood vessels). Targeted therapy is often used in cancers with known driver mutations or molecular targets.

6. **Hormone Therapy**: Hormone therapy is used to block or suppress hormone receptors in hormone-sensitive cancers such as breast and prostate cancer. It may involve medications that inhibit hormone production, block

hormone receptors, or interfere with hormone signaling pathways.

7. **Stem Cell Transplantation**: Stem cell transplantation, also known as bone marrow transplantation, involves replacing diseased or damaged bone marrow with healthy stem cells to restore normal blood cell production. It is commonly used in the treatment of leukemia, lymphoma, and other hematologic malignancies.

Challenges and Advances in Cancer Treatment

Despite significant progress in cancer treatment, several challenges remain, including treatment resistance, toxicity, recurrence, and metastasis. Researchers continue to explore novel therapeutic approaches and innovative strategies to overcome these challenges and improve patient outcomes.

Recent advances in cancer treatment include:

1. **Precision Medicine**: Precision medicine, also known as personalized or genomic medicine, aims to tailor cancer treatment to individual patients based on their unique genetic profile, tumor characteristics, and other factors. This approach enables more targeted and effective therapies while minimizing adverse effects.

2. **Liquid Biopsies**: Liquid biopsies involve analyzing circulating tumor cells, cell-free DNA, RNA, proteins, and other

biomarkers in blood or other bodily fluids to detect cancer, monitor disease progression, and guide treatment decisions. Liquid biopsies offer a non-invasive and real-time approach to cancer diagnosis and monitoring.

3. **Immunogenomics**: Immunogenomics integrates genomics and immunology to understand how genetic variations influence immune responses to cancer and identify novel immunotherapeutic targets. By elucidating the complex interactions between tumors and the immune system, immunogenomics informs the development of personalized immunotherapies.

4. **Nanomedicine**: Nanomedicine involves the use of nanoparticles and nanotechnology-based delivery systems to target cancer cells with precision, enhance drug delivery, and minimize systemic toxicity. Nanomedicine holds promise for improving the efficacy and safety of cancer treatments, including chemotherapy and targeted therapy.

In conclusion, understanding the causes, types, and conventional treatments of cancer is essential for effectively combating this complex and heterogeneous disease. While conventional therapies such as surgery, chemotherapy, radiation therapy, immunotherapy, targeted therapy, and hormone therapy remain cornerstone modalities in cancer treatment, ongoing research and technological advancements offer hope for more personalized, precise, and innovative approaches to cancer care.

CHAPTER THREE

The Role of Herbal Medicine in Cancer Management

Herbal medicine, also known as botanical medicine or phytotherapy, has been utilized for centuries across diverse cultures as a primary or complementary approach to managing various health conditions, including cancer. In recent years, there has been growing interest in the potential role of herbal medicine in cancer management, driven by the need for effective and less toxic treatment options. Herbal remedies derived from plants offer a rich source of bioactive compounds with diverse pharmacological properties, including anticancer effects. Understanding the role of herbal medicine in cancer management involves exploring its mechanisms of action, evidence base, clinical applications, and considerations for integration into comprehensive treatment protocols.

Mechanisms of Action

Herbal medicines exert their effects through a multitude of mechanisms that may target various aspects of cancer development and progression. Some of the key mechanisms of action include:

1. **Antioxidant Activity**: Many herbs contain compounds with potent antioxidant properties, such as polyphenols,

flavonoids, and carotenoids. These antioxidants help neutralize reactive oxygen species (ROS) and reduce oxidative stress, which is implicated in cancer initiation and promotion.

2. **Anti-inflammatory Effects**: Chronic inflammation plays a critical role in cancer development by promoting cell proliferation, angiogenesis, and metastasis. Herbal remedies with anti-inflammatory properties can modulate inflammatory pathways and suppress tumor-associated inflammation.

3. **Immune Modulation**: Herbal medicines can modulate immune function by enhancing innate and adaptive immune responses against cancer cells. Certain herbs stimulate the activity of immune cells such as natural killer (NK) cells, cytotoxic T cells, and macrophages, leading to enhanced tumor surveillance and elimination.

4. **Apoptosis Induction**: Apoptosis, or programmed cell death, is a fundamental process that regulates cell turnover and eliminates damaged or abnormal cells, including cancer cells. Herbal compounds can induce apoptosis in cancer cells by activating intrinsic or extrinsic apoptotic pathways.

5. **Cell Cycle Regulation**: Dysregulation of the cell cycle, leading to uncontrolled cell proliferation, is a hallmark of cancer. Herbal medicines can modulate cell cycle checkpoints and

regulatory proteins involved in cell division, thereby inhibiting tumor growth and promoting cell cycle arrest.

6. **Angiogenesis Inhibition**: Angiogenesis, the formation of new blood vessels, is essential for tumor growth and metastasis. Herbal compounds can inhibit angiogenesis by targeting pro-angiogenic factors such as vascular endothelial growth factor (VEGF), thereby depriving tumors of blood supply and nutrient delivery.

7. **Anti-metastatic Activity**: Metastasis, the spread of cancer cells to distant sites, is a major cause of mortality in cancer patients. Herbal medicines may possess anti-metastatic properties by inhibiting cell migration, invasion, adhesion, and epithelial-mesenchymal transition (EMT), thereby impeding the metastatic cascade.

Evidence Base

While traditional herbal remedies have been used for centuries in cancer management, their efficacy and safety have been the subject of increasing scientific scrutiny. A growing body of preclinical and clinical research has investigated the anticancer properties of various herbs and plant-derived compounds, providing insights into their mechanisms of action and potential therapeutic applications.

1. **Preclinical Studies**: Preclinical studies conducted in laboratory settings, including in vitro cell culture and animal

models, have demonstrated the anticancer effects of numerous herbal extracts, fractions, and isolated compounds. These studies provide valuable insights into the molecular targets and pathways modulated by herbal medicines and serve as a basis for further investigation.

2. **Clinical Trials**: Clinical trials evaluating the efficacy and safety of herbal medicines in cancer patients have yielded mixed results. While some trials have reported beneficial effects such as tumor regression, symptom relief, improved quality of life, and prolonged survival, others have shown no significant difference compared to placebo or standard treatment. Challenges in clinical trial design, including heterogeneous patient populations, variable herbal formulations, limited sample sizes, and lack of standardized endpoints, contribute to the variability in outcomes.

3. **Meta-analyses and Systematic Reviews**: Meta-analyses and systematic reviews provide a comprehensive synthesis of existing evidence from multiple studies to assess the overall efficacy and safety of herbal medicines in cancer management. While some meta-analyses support the use of certain herbal remedies as adjunctive therapies for specific types of cancer, others highlight the need for further well-designed clinical trials to confirm their benefits.

Clinical Applications

Herbal medicine can be integrated into cancer management in various ways, depending on factors such as cancer type, stage, patient preferences, and treatment goals. Some common clinical applications of herbal medicine in cancer management include:

1. **Adjunctive Therapy**: Herbal remedies may be used as adjuncts to conventional cancer treatments such as surgery, chemotherapy, radiation therapy, and immunotherapy to enhance their efficacy, reduce side effects, and improve overall outcomes. Herbal formulations tailored to individual patient needs may target specific aspects of cancer biology or support overall health and well-being.

2. **Symptom Management**: Herbal medicines can alleviate cancer-related symptoms and side effects of treatment, including pain, nausea, vomiting, fatigue, anxiety, depression, insomnia, and loss of appetite. Herbal formulations with analgesic, antiemetic, anxiolytic, sedative, and adaptogenic properties may provide symptomatic relief and improve quality of life.

3. **Supportive Care**: Herbal remedies can support the body's natural healing processes and resilience during cancer treatment and recovery. Herbal formulations rich in vitamins, minerals, antioxidants, and phytonutrients may enhance immune function, promote tissue repair, and

mitigate the effects of stress, malnutrition, and toxicity associated with cancer therapy.

4. **Prevention and Risk Reduction**: Herbal medicine may play a role in cancer prevention and risk reduction by addressing modifiable risk factors, promoting healthy lifestyle habits, and enhancing the body's defense mechanisms against carcinogenesis. Herbal formulations with chemopreventive, antioxidant, anti-inflammatory, and immunomodulatory properties may help reduce the incidence of certain cancers and improve overall health outcomes.

Considerations for Integration

Integration of herbal medicine into cancer management requires careful consideration of several factors to ensure safety, efficacy, and patient-centered care:

1. **Evidence-Based Practice**: Clinicians should base their recommendations on the best available evidence from scientific research, clinical experience, and patient preferences. While traditional knowledge and anecdotal evidence may inform herbal practice, they should be complemented by rigorous scientific inquiry and critical appraisal of the literature.

2. **Interdisciplinary Collaboration**: Collaboration between healthcare providers, including oncologists, herbalists, naturopathic physicians, integrative oncologists,

pharmacists, and other allied health professionals, is essential for comprehensive cancer care. Interdisciplinary teams can facilitate communication, coordination, and integration of herbal medicine with conventional treatments, ensuring optimal patient outcomes and safety.

3. **Individualized Treatment**: Cancer management should be tailored to individual patient needs, preferences, and circumstances. Herbal formulations should be personalized based on factors such as cancer type, stage, prognosis, comorbidities, concurrent medications, allergies, dietary habits, lifestyle factors, and psychosocial support systems.

4. **Quality Assurance**: Quality assurance and safety of herbal products are paramount to minimize the risk of contamination, adulteration, mislabeling, and variability in potency and efficacy. Clinicians should recommend reputable suppliers that adhere to Good Manufacturing Practices (GMP), provide transparent product labeling, conduct rigorous quality control testing, and ensure sustainability and ethical sourcing of botanical ingredients.

5. **Patient Education and Empowerment**: Patient education and empowerment are essential for informed decision-making, adherence to treatment protocols, and self-care practices. Clinicians should provide accurate, balanced, and culturally sensitive information about the benefits, risks, and

limitations of herbal medicine, as well as strategies for integrating herbal therapies into cancer management plans.

6. **Monitoring and Follow-up**: Regular monitoring and follow-up are necessary to evaluate the efficacy, safety, and tolerability of herbal medicine, assess disease progression, manage treatment-related side effects, and make appropriate adjustments to the treatment plan as needed. Clinicians should establish clear communication channels with patients and encourage open dialogue about their experiences, concerns, and goals throughout the cancer journey.

In conclusion, herbal medicine plays a multifaceted role in cancer management, offering potential benefits as adjunctive therapies for symptom management, supportive care, prevention, and risk reduction. While the evidence base for herbal medicine in cancer management continues to evolve, integration of herbal therapies into comprehensive treatment protocols requires a patient-centered approach, interdisciplinary collaboration, evidence-based practice, quality assurance, patient education, and ongoing monitoring and follow-up. By harnessing the therapeutic potential of herbal remedies in conjunction with conventional cancer treatments, clinicians can optimize patient outcomes and improve quality of life for individuals affected by cancer.

CHAPTER FOUR

Dr. Barbara's Principles of Herbal Healing and Cancer Prevention

Dr. Barbara's principles of herbal healing and cancer prevention are rooted in a holistic approach that emphasizes the importance of addressing the underlying causes of disease, supporting the body's innate healing mechanisms, and promoting overall health and well-being. Through personalized herbal protocols, lifestyle modifications, and preventive strategies, Dr. Barbara aims to empower individuals to take an active role in maintaining optimal health and reducing the risk of cancer.

1. Holistic Assessment and Individualized Care

Dr. Barbara believes in treating the whole person, not just the disease. Each individual is unique, with distinct genetic predispositions, lifestyle factors, environmental exposures, and health challenges. Therefore, Dr. Barbara conducts a thorough holistic assessment that takes into account various aspects of a person's physical, emotional, mental, and spiritual health.

By understanding the interconnectedness of body, mind, and spirit, Dr. Barbara tailors her herbal healing and cancer prevention strategies to address the specific needs, preferences, and goals of each individual. This personalized approach ensures that treatment plans are not only effective but also empowering and sustainable, fostering a sense of ownership and partnership in the healing process.

2. Emphasis on Prevention and Lifestyle Modification

Prevention is at the core of Dr. Barbara's approach to health and wellness. Rather than waiting for disease to manifest, Dr. Barbara focuses on proactive measures to optimize health, prevent illness, and promote longevity. She emphasizes the importance of lifestyle modification, including dietary changes, regular physical activity, stress management, adequate sleep, and avoidance of harmful habits such as smoking and excessive alcohol consumption.

In the context of cancer prevention, Dr. Barbara educates individuals about modifiable risk factors and empowers them to make informed choices that reduce their likelihood of developing cancer. This may involve adopting a plant-based diet rich in fruits, vegetables, whole grains, and legumes; minimizing exposure to environmental toxins and carcinogens; maintaining a healthy body weight; practicing sun safety; and participating in regular cancer screenings and health assessments.

3. Healing Power of Nature and Herbal Medicine

Dr. Barbara harnesses the healing power of nature and herbal medicine to promote health, prevent disease, and support the body's self-healing mechanisms. Plants have been used for millennia in traditional healing systems around the world for their medicinal properties and therapeutic benefits. Herbal remedies contain a myriad of bioactive compounds, including phytochemicals, antioxidants, vitamins, minerals, and essential oils, which exert multifaceted effects on the body.

Dr. Barbara selects specific herbs and botanicals based on their traditional uses, scientific evidence, and individualized needs to create customized herbal formulations tailored to each person's unique constitution and health goals. These herbal protocols may include teas, tinctures, capsules, extracts, poultices, or topical preparations, depending on the desired therapeutic outcomes and mode of administration.

4. Support for Immune Function and Detoxification

A robust immune system is essential for protecting the body against infections, toxins, and cancerous cells. Dr. Barbara emphasizes the importance of immune support as a cornerstone of cancer prevention and holistic health maintenance. Herbal remedies with immunomodulatory properties can enhance immune function, stimulate immune surveillance, and promote the body's ability to recognize and eliminate abnormal cells before they develop into cancer.

Furthermore, Dr. Barbara recognizes the role of detoxification in promoting optimal health and preventing disease. Environmental toxins, pollutants, heavy metals, pesticides, and other xenobiotics can accumulate in the body over time, impairing cellular function, disrupting hormonal balance, and increasing the risk of cancer and other chronic diseases. Herbal therapies that support liver function, enhance detoxification pathways, and facilitate elimination of toxins can help maintain cellular integrity and reduce the burden on the body's detoxification organs.

5. Empowerment Through Education and Self-Care

Central to Dr. Barbara's philosophy is the belief in empowering individuals to take control of their health through education, self-awareness, and self-care practices. She provides comprehensive education about the principles of herbal healing, cancer prevention strategies, and lifestyle modifications, equipping individuals with the knowledge and tools they need to make informed decisions and advocate for their own well-being.

Dr. Barbara encourages self-care practices that promote mindfulness, resilience, and inner balance, such as meditation, yoga, tai chi, breathwork, journaling, and creative expression. These practices not only help manage stress and enhance emotional well-being but also strengthen the mind-body connection and cultivate a sense of harmony and wholeness.

In conclusion, Dr. Barbara's principles of herbal healing and cancer prevention embody a holistic and integrative approach to health and wellness. By addressing the root causes of disease, emphasizing prevention and lifestyle modification, harnessing the healing power of nature and herbal medicine, supporting immune function and detoxification, and empowering individuals through education and self-care, Dr. Barbara aims to promote optimal health, vitality, and resilience while reducing the risk of cancer and other chronic illnesses.

CHAPTER FIVE

The Importance of Nutrition and Lifestyle in Cancer Prevention and Treatment

Nutrition and lifestyle factors play a significant role in cancer prevention and treatment. Mounting evidence suggests that dietary choices, physical activity, weight management, and other lifestyle behaviors can influence cancer risk, prognosis, and overall health outcomes. Adopting a healthy lifestyle that includes a balanced diet, regular exercise, stress management, adequate sleep, and avoidance of harmful habits can help reduce the incidence of cancer, enhance treatment efficacy, improve quality of life, and promote long-term survivorship.

1. Dietary Patterns and Cancer Risk

A growing body of research supports the role of dietary patterns in modulating cancer risk. Diets rich in fruits, vegetables, whole grains, legumes, nuts, seeds, and lean proteins are associated with a lower risk of developing certain types of cancer, including colorectal, breast, prostate, lung, and stomach cancer. These foods are abundant in vitamins, minerals, antioxidants, fiber, and phytochemicals, which have protective effects against carcinogenesis by neutralizing free radicals, reducing inflammation, and promoting DNA repair and apoptosis.

Conversely, diets high in processed and red meats, sugary beverages, refined carbohydrates, saturated fats, and trans fats are linked to an increased risk of cancer and other chronic diseases. These foods may promote inflammation, insulin resistance, oxidative stress, and dysbiosis, creating an environment conducive to tumor growth, angiogenesis, and metastasis.

2. Phytochemicals and Cancer Prevention

Phytochemicals are bioactive compounds found in plants that have been shown to possess anticancer properties. These compounds, including polyphenols, flavonoids, carotenoids, glucosinolates, and lignans, exert diverse effects on cellular pathways involved in cancer development and progression. For example, resveratrol in grapes and red wine, curcumin in turmeric, epigallocatechin gallate (EGCG) in green tea, and sulforaphane in cruciferous vegetables have been studied for their chemopreventive effects against various types of cancer.

Phytochemical-rich foods act synergistically to inhibit carcinogenesis through antioxidant, anti-inflammatory, anti-proliferative, anti-angiogenic, and pro-apoptotic mechanisms. Incorporating a wide variety of colorful fruits, vegetables, herbs, and spices into the diet can provide a diverse array of phytochemicals with complementary and overlapping effects, thereby maximizing their potential benefits for cancer prevention and overall health.

3. Physical Activity and Cancer Prevention

Regular physical activity is associated with a reduced risk of developing certain types of cancer, including colon, breast, endometrial, and prostate cancer. Exercise has numerous physiological effects that contribute to cancer prevention, such as improving insulin sensitivity, reducing chronic inflammation, enhancing immune function, promoting hormonal balance, and facilitating weight management.

Furthermore, physical activity can directly inhibit tumor growth and progression by modulating signaling pathways involved in cell proliferation, apoptosis, angiogenesis, and metastasis. Exercise-induced changes in hormone levels, cytokine profiles, and metabolic pathways may create an inhospitable microenvironment for cancer cells, making them more susceptible to immune surveillance and elimination.

4. Weight Management and Cancer Risk Reduction

Excess body weight, particularly abdominal obesity, is a significant risk factor for several types of cancer, including colorectal, breast, endometrial, kidney, pancreatic, and esophageal cancer. Obesity is associated with chronic low-grade inflammation, insulin resistance, dyslipidemia, altered hormone levels, and oxidative stress, which contribute to carcinogenesis and tumor progression.

Maintaining a healthy weight through a combination of balanced nutrition, regular physical activity, and lifestyle modifications is essential for reducing cancer risk and improving overall health outcomes. Even modest reductions in body weight and waist circumference can have significant benefits in terms of cancer prevention, metabolic health, and quality of life.

5. Stress Management and Psychosocial Support

Chronic stress and negative emotional states such as anxiety, depression, and social isolation have been linked to an increased risk of cancer recurrence, progression, and mortality. Stress-induced changes in neuroendocrine, immune, and inflammatory pathways may promote tumor growth, angiogenesis, and metastasis, while compromising immune surveillance and antitumor immunity.

Incorporating stress management techniques such as mindfulness meditation, yoga, deep breathing exercises, progressive muscle relaxation, and cognitive-behavioral therapy into daily life can help reduce stress levels, improve coping skills, and enhance emotional well-being. Social support networks, peer groups, and counseling services can also provide valuable resources for individuals navigating the challenges of cancer diagnosis, treatment, and survivorship.

6. Avoidance of Harmful Habits

Certain lifestyle habits, such as tobacco use, excessive alcohol consumption, and exposure to environmental toxins, are known carcinogens that significantly increase the risk of developing cancer. Tobacco smoke contains over 7,000 chemicals, including carcinogens such as benzene, formaldehyde, and polycyclic aromatic hydrocarbons, which can damage DNA, promote inflammation, and induce malignant transformation.

Similarly, heavy alcohol consumption is associated with an increased risk of several types of cancer, including oral, throat, esophageal, liver, breast, and colorectal cancer. Alcohol can disrupt hormone levels, impair DNA repair mechanisms, and generate oxidative stress, contributing to tumor initiation and progression.

Avoiding tobacco use, limiting alcohol intake, and minimizing exposure to environmental carcinogens are essential for reducing cancer risk and optimizing overall health outcomes. Smoking cessation programs, alcohol moderation strategies, and environmental health initiatives can provide support and resources for individuals seeking to adopt healthier habits and minimize their cancer risk.

In conclusion, nutrition and lifestyle factors play a crucial role in cancer prevention and treatment. By adopting a balanced diet, engaging in regular physical activity, maintaining a healthy weight, managing stress effectively, avoiding harmful habits, and seeking psychosocial support when needed, individuals can empower themselves to reduce their cancer risk, enhance treatment outcomes, and improve their overall quality of life. Integrating these lifestyle interventions into comprehensive cancer care plans can complement conventional therapies and promote holistic well-being for individuals affected by cancer.

CHAPTER SIX

Selecting the Right Herbs for Cancer Healing: Dr. Barbara's Recommendations

Dr. Barbara's approach to selecting herbs for cancer healing is rooted in a holistic understanding of the individual's unique constitution, health status, treatment goals, and preferences. By integrating traditional knowledge, scientific evidence, and clinical experience, Dr. Barbara customizes herbal protocols that address the multifaceted aspects of cancer, including tumor biology, immune function, symptom management, and overall well-being. Here are some of Dr. Barbara's recommendations for selecting the right herbs for cancer healing:

1. Comprehensive Assessment

Before recommending specific herbs, Dr. Barbara conducts a comprehensive assessment of the individual's health history, current symptoms, treatment regimen, dietary habits, lifestyle factors, and goals for cancer healing. This holistic approach allows Dr. Barbara to identify underlying imbalances, nutritional deficiencies, toxic exposures, and other factors that may influence cancer progression and treatment response.

2. Individualized Formulations

Dr. Barbara believes in the importance of individualized herbal formulations tailored to each person's unique needs and preferences. Rather than employing a one-size-fits-all approach, Dr. Barbara carefully selects herbs based on their therapeutic properties, compatibility with the individual's constitution, and potential interactions with other medications or treatments.

For example, individuals undergoing chemotherapy or radiation therapy may benefit from herbs with cytoprotective, immune-modulating, and antiemetic properties to alleviate treatment-related side effects and enhance tolerance to therapy. Similarly, patients with hormone-sensitive cancers may benefit from herbs that regulate hormonal balance and support endocrine function.

3. Evidence-Based Herbal Medicine

Dr. Barbara incorporates evidence-based herbal medicine into her practice, drawing upon scientific research, clinical trials, and traditional wisdom to inform her recommendations. While traditional herbal knowledge provides valuable insights into the therapeutic properties of medicinal plants, Dr. Barbara emphasizes the importance of rigorous scientific inquiry and critical appraisal of the literature to ensure the safety, efficacy, and quality of herbal remedies.

Herbs with well-established anticancer properties supported by scientific evidence may include:

- **Turmeric (Curcuma longa)**: Known for its potent anti-inflammatory, antioxidant, and anticancer properties, curcumin, the active compound in turmeric, has been studied for its potential therapeutic effects in various types of cancer, including breast, colorectal, prostate, and pancreatic cancer.

- **Green Tea (Camellia sinensis)**: Rich in polyphenols such as epigallocatechin gallate (EGCG), green tea exhibits antioxidant, anti-inflammatory, and anticancer activities that may help inhibit tumor growth, angiogenesis, and metastasis in cancers such as breast, prostate, lung, and colorectal cancer.

- **Reishi Mushroom (Ganoderma lucidum)**: Revered for its immune-modulating, anti-inflammatory, and antitumor properties, reishi mushroom has been used in traditional medicine to support immune function, enhance vitality, and improve overall health. Research suggests that reishi mushroom extracts may have potential therapeutic benefits in cancer prevention and treatment.

- **Astragalus (Astragalus membranaceus)**: Known as an adaptogenic herb, astragalus supports immune function, enhances resilience to stress, and promotes overall vitality. Studies have shown that astragalus extracts may stimulate immune cell activity and exert antitumor effects in certain types of cancer.

4. Safety and Quality Assurance

Dr. Barbara prioritizes safety and quality assurance when selecting herbs for cancer healing. She recommends reputable suppliers that adhere to Good Manufacturing Practices (GMP), conduct rigorous quality control testing, and provide transparent product labeling to ensure the purity, potency, and integrity of herbal products.

Additionally, Dr. Barbara educates individuals about potential herb-drug interactions, contraindications, and precautions to minimize the risk of adverse effects and optimize therapeutic outcomes. Open communication, informed consent, and ongoing monitoring are essential components of Dr. Barbara's patient-centered approach to herbal healing.

5. Integrative Approach

Dr. Barbara advocates for an integrative approach to cancer healing that combines the best of conventional and complementary therapies to optimize patient outcomes and promote holistic well-being. Herbal medicine can complement conventional cancer treatments such as surgery, chemotherapy, radiation therapy, immunotherapy, and hormone therapy by addressing side effects, enhancing treatment efficacy, and supporting the body's natural healing processes.

Furthermore, Dr. Barbara emphasizes the importance of lifestyle modifications, dietary changes, stress management techniques, and psychosocial support as integral components of cancer healing. By addressing the physical, emotional, mental, and spiritual dimensions of health, Dr. Barbara empowers individuals to cultivate resilience, enhance quality of life, and thrive beyond cancer.

In conclusion, selecting the right herbs for cancer healing requires a personalized and evidence-based approach that takes into account the individual's unique needs, preferences, and circumstances. By integrating traditional knowledge, scientific research, and clinical expertise, Dr. Barbara provides tailored herbal protocols that support the body's innate healing mechanisms, promote overall well-being, and empower individuals on their journey to healing and wholeness.

CHAPTER SEVEN

Herbal remedies and formulations

Herbal remedies and formulations can play a complementary role in supporting conventional cancer treatments and addressing symptoms associated with specific types of cancer. Dr. Barbara recommends a personalized approach to herbal medicine, taking into account the individual's unique constitution, cancer diagnosis, treatment plan, and overall health status. While herbal remedies should not be used as a substitute for conventional cancer therapies, they can enhance quality of life, alleviate treatment-related side effects, and support the body's natural healing processes. Here are some herbal remedies and formulations that may be beneficial for specific types of cancer:

1. Breast Cancer:

- **Turmeric (Curcuma longa)**: Known for its anti-inflammatory and antioxidant properties, curcumin, the active compound in turmeric, may help inhibit the growth and spread of breast cancer cells and enhance the efficacy of chemotherapy and radiation therapy.

- **Green Tea (Camellia sinensis)**: Rich in polyphenols such as EGCG, green tea has been studied for its potential chemopreventive and anticancer effects in breast cancer, including inhibition of tumor growth and metastasis.

- **Soy Isoflavones**: Soy foods and supplements containing isoflavones such as genistein and daidzein may exert protective effects against breast cancer by modulating estrogen metabolism and hormone receptor signaling pathways.

2. Prostate Cancer:

- **Saw Palmetto (Serenoa repens)**: Saw palmetto extract is commonly used to support prostate health and alleviate urinary symptoms associated with benign prostatic hyperplasia (BPH). Some studies suggest that saw palmetto may also have antiandrogenic effects that could be beneficial for prostate cancer.

- **Stinging Nettle (Urtica dioica)**: Nettle root extract has been traditionally used to relieve urinary symptoms and support prostate health. It may help reduce inflammation, inhibit the growth of prostate cancer cells, and improve urinary flow.

- **Pygeum (Pygeum africanum)**: Pygeum bark extract has been shown to improve urinary symptoms and quality of life in men with BPH. It may also have anti-inflammatory and anti-proliferative effects that could be relevant for prostate cancer.

3. Colorectal Cancer:

- **Aloe Vera (Aloe barbadensis)**: Aloe vera gel contains bioactive compounds such as polysaccharides, anthraquinones, and flavonoids that have anti-inflammatory, antioxidant, and immunomodulatory properties. Some studies suggest that aloe vera may help reduce inflammation, promote wound healing, and inhibit the growth of colorectal cancer cells.

- **Ginger (Zingiber officinale)**: Ginger root contains gingerols and other bioactive compounds that possess anti-inflammatory, antioxidant, and anticancer properties. Ginger may help alleviate nausea, vomiting, and gastrointestinal symptoms associated with colorectal cancer and its treatment.

- **Boswellia (Boswellia serrata)**: Boswellia resin extract contains boswellic acids, which have anti-inflammatory and anticancer effects. Boswellia may help reduce inflammation, pain, and tumor growth in colorectal cancer.

4. Lung Cancer:

- **Echinacea (Echinacea spp.)**: Echinacea root extract has immune-modulating properties that may enhance immune function and improve resistance to respiratory infections in lung cancer patients.

- **Licorice (Glycyrrhiza glabra)**: Licorice root contains glycyrrhizin and other bioactive compounds that have anti-inflammatory, antiviral, and immunomodulatory effects. Licorice may help reduce inflammation, cough, and respiratory symptoms associated with lung cancer and its treatment.

- **Mullein (Verbascum thapsus)**: Mullein leaf extract has demulcent and expectorant properties that can soothe respiratory irritation, alleviate cough, and promote respiratory health in lung cancer patients.

5. Skin Cancer:

- **Green Tea (Camellia sinensis)**: Topical application of green tea extracts containing EGCG may help protect the skin from UV-induced damage, reduce inflammation, and inhibit the growth of skin cancer cells.

- **Aloe Vera (Aloe barbadensis)**: Aloe vera gel has cooling and soothing properties that can relieve sunburn, inflammation, and irritation associated with skin cancer and its treatment.

- **Calendula (Calendula officinalis)**: Calendula flower extract has anti-inflammatory, antimicrobial, and wound-healing properties that can promote skin repair and alleviate skin irritation in skin cancer patients.

It's important to consult with a qualified healthcare practitioner before using herbal remedies, especially if you are undergoing cancer treatment or have other medical conditions. Herbal remedies may interact with medications or treatments and may not be suitable for everyone. Additionally, ensure that herbal products are sourced from reputable suppliers and are of high quality and purity. Integrating herbal remedies into a comprehensive cancer care plan can provide additional support and improve quality of life for individuals affected by cancer.

CHAPTER EIGHT

Integrating herbal medicine with conventional cancer therapies

Integrating herbal medicine with conventional cancer therapies involves a collaborative and holistic approach that combines the best of both worlds to optimize patient outcomes, enhance quality of life, and promote holistic well-being. While conventional cancer therapies such as surgery, chemotherapy, radiation therapy, immunotherapy, and hormone therapy are often the primary treatment modalities for cancer, herbal medicine can play a complementary role in supporting the body's natural healing processes, alleviating treatment-related side effects, and improving overall health outcomes. Here are some key considerations for integrating herbal medicine with conventional cancer therapies:

1. Multidisciplinary Collaboration: Effective integration of herbal medicine with conventional cancer therapies requires collaboration between healthcare providers from different disciplines, including oncologists, herbalists, naturopathic physicians, integrative oncologists, pharmacists, and other allied health professionals. Multidisciplinary teams can facilitate communication, coordination, and integration of treatment plans, ensuring that patient care is comprehensive, cohesive, and patient-centered.

2. Patient-Centered Care: Central to the integration of herbal medicine with conventional cancer therapies is a patient-centered approach that takes into account the individual's unique needs, preferences, values, and treatment goals. Healthcare providers should engage patients in shared decision-making, provide accurate information about treatment options, and empower them to make informed choices that align with their beliefs and priorities.

3. Evidence-Informed Practice: While traditional herbal knowledge provides valuable insights into the therapeutic properties of medicinal plants, evidence-informed practice relies on scientific research, clinical trials, and empirical evidence to guide decision-making and ensure the safety, efficacy, and quality of herbal remedies. Healthcare providers should stay updated on the latest research findings and critically appraise the literature to inform their recommendations and treatment protocols.

4. Complementary Supportive Care: Herbal medicine can complement conventional cancer therapies by providing supportive care that addresses symptom management, side effect mitigation, and overall well-being. Herbal remedies may help alleviate nausea, vomiting, fatigue, pain, anxiety, depression, insomnia, and other treatment-related side effects, improving quality of life and treatment adherence.

5. Individualized Herbal Protocols: Herbal protocols should be individualized based on the patient's cancer type, stage, treatment regimen, health status, dietary habits, lifestyle factors, and preferences. Herbalists and healthcare providers can customize herbal formulations to target specific symptoms, support organ function, enhance immune function, and promote overall health and vitality.

6. Safety and Quality Assurance: Safety and quality assurance are paramount when integrating herbal medicine with conventional cancer therapies. Healthcare providers should recommend reputable suppliers that adhere to Good Manufacturing Practices (GMP), conduct rigorous quality control testing, and provide transparent product labeling to ensure the purity, potency, and integrity of herbal products. Patients should be educated about potential herb-drug interactions, contraindications, and precautions to minimize the risk of adverse effects and optimize therapeutic outcomes.

7. Ongoing Monitoring and Follow-Up: Regular monitoring and follow-up are essential to evaluate the efficacy, safety, and tolerability of herbal medicine, assess treatment response, manage side effects, and make appropriate adjustments to the treatment plan as needed. Healthcare providers should establish clear communication channels with patients and encourage open dialogue about their experiences, concerns, and goals throughout the cancer journey.

In conclusion, integrating herbal medicine with conventional cancer therapies involves a collaborative, patient-centered, and evidence-informed approach that prioritizes safety, efficacy, and quality of care. By harnessing the synergistic benefits of both modalities, healthcare providers can optimize patient outcomes, improve quality of life, and promote holistic well-being for individuals affected by cancer.

CHAPTER NINE

MANAGING TREATMENT SYMTHOMS

Herbal protocols can be valuable adjuncts to conventional cancer therapies for managing symptoms and side effects, enhancing quality of life, and supporting overall well-being during treatment and recovery. While herbal remedies should not replace standard medical care, they can complement conventional interventions by addressing common symptoms and side effects associated with cancer and its treatments. Here are some herbal protocols for managing cancer symptoms and side effects:

1. Nausea and Vomiting:

- **Ginger (Zingiber officinale)**: Ginger is well-known for its anti-nausea properties and can be consumed as fresh ginger root, ginger tea, or ginger supplements to alleviate nausea and vomiting associated with chemotherapy, radiation therapy, or surgery.

- **Peppermint (Mentha piperita)**: Peppermint tea or peppermint oil may help relieve nausea and promote digestion, making it useful for managing chemotherapy-induced nausea and vomiting.

- **Chamomile (Matricaria chamomilla)**: Chamomile tea has calming and anti-inflammatory effects that may help reduce nausea and soothe the digestive tract.

2. Fatigue:

- **Panax Ginseng (Panax ginseng)**: Ginseng root is an adaptogenic herb that can help improve energy levels, reduce fatigue, and enhance physical and mental performance during cancer treatment.

- **Rhodiola (Rhodiola rosea)**: Rhodiola root extract has adaptogenic properties that can increase resilience to stress, improve endurance, and alleviate fatigue associated with cancer and its treatments.

- **Ashwagandha (Withaniasomnifera)**: Ashwagandha root is an adaptogenic herb that may help reduce fatigue, enhance vitality, and improve overall well-being in cancer patients.

3. Pain Management:

- **Turmeric (Curcuma longa)**: Curcumin, the active compound in turmeric, has anti-inflammatory and analgesic properties that may help reduce pain and inflammation associated with cancer and its treatments.

- **White Willow Bark (Salix alba)**: White willow bark contains salicin, a natural compound with pain-relieving and anti-inflammatory effects similar to aspirin. It may help alleviate mild to moderate pain in cancer patients.

- **Cannabis (Cannabis spp.)**: Cannabis-derived products containing cannabinoids such as THC and CBD have been used to manage cancer-related pain, neuropathy, and inflammation. However, it's important to use cannabis products under medical supervision due to potential side effects and legal considerations.

4. Anxiety and Depression:

- **Lavender (Lavandula angustifolia)**: Lavender essential oil or lavender tea may help reduce anxiety, promote relaxation, and improve sleep quality in cancer patients.

- **Passionflower (Passiflora incarnata)**: Passionflower extract has calming and sedative properties that can help alleviate anxiety, insomnia, and restlessness in cancer patients.

- **St. John's Wort (Hypericum perforatum)**: St. John's Wort is a herbal remedy that has been studied for its antidepressant effects and may help improve mood and emotional well-being in cancer patients experiencing depression.

5. Digestive Issues:

- **Peppermint (Mentha piperita)**: Peppermint tea or peppermint oil may help relieve gastrointestinal symptoms such as bloating, gas, indigestion, and abdominal discomfort.

- **Licorice (Glycyrrhiza glabra)**: Licorice root extract can help soothe the digestive tract, reduce inflammation, and promote gastric mucosal protection, making it useful for managing gastritis and acid reflux.

- **Marshmallow Root (Althaea officinalis)**: Marshmallow root contains mucilage, a soothing gel-like substance that can coat the digestive tract and alleviate irritation, inflammation, and discomfort associated with conditions such as gastritis, esophagitis, and peptic ulcers.

6. Immune Support:

- **Astragalus (Astragalus membranaceus)**: Astragalus root is an adaptogenic herb that can help support immune function, enhance vitality, and improve resistance to infections during cancer treatment.

- **Medicinal Mushrooms (e.g., Reishi, Shiitake, Maitake)**: Medicinal mushrooms contain beta-glucans and other bioactive compounds that can modulate immune function, increase white blood cell activity, and promote overall health and resilience.

- **Echinacea (Echinacea spp.)**: Echinacea root extract has immune-modulating properties that may help enhance immune response and reduce the risk of infections in cancer patients undergoing treatment.

7. Sleep Disturbances:

- **Valerian (Valeriana officinalis)**: Valerian root extract has sedative and anxiolytic properties that can help promote relaxation, improve sleep quality, and alleviate insomnia in cancer patients.

- **Passionflower (Passiflora incarnata)**: Passionflower extract may help calm the mind, reduce anxiety, and induce restful sleep in cancer patients experiencing sleep disturbances.

- **Lemon Balm (Melissa officinalis)**: Lemon balm tea or lemon balm essential oil may help reduce anxiety, promote relaxation, and improve sleep patterns in cancer patients.

It's important to consult with a qualified healthcare practitioner, such as a naturopathic doctor, herbalist, or integrative oncologist, before using herbal remedies, especially if you are undergoing cancer treatment or have other medical conditions. Herbal remedies may interact with medications or treatments and may not be suitable for everyone. Additionally, ensure that herbal products are sourced from reputable suppliers and are of high quality and purity. Integrating herbal protocols into a comprehensive cancer care plan can provide additional support and improve quality of life for individuals affected by cancer.

CHAPTER TEN

Empowering Yourself Through Herbal Medicine: Practical Steps for Cancer Patients and Caregivers

Navigating a cancer diagnosis and treatment journey can be overwhelming, but empowering yourself through herbal medicine can provide valuable tools for managing symptoms, supporting overall well-being, and enhancing quality of life. While herbal medicine should not replace conventional cancer therapies, it can complement standard treatments and empower individuals to take an active role in their healing process. Here are some practical steps for cancer patients and caregivers to incorporate herbal medicine into their care:

1. Educate Yourself: Take the time to learn about herbal medicine, including common herbs, their therapeutic properties, potential benefits, and safety considerations. There are many reputable resources available, including books, websites, online courses, and educational materials from trusted organizations.

2. Consult with Qualified Professionals: Work with qualified healthcare practitioners who have expertise in herbal medicine, such as naturopathic doctors, herbalists, or integrative oncologists. They can provide personalized recommendations, guidance on herb selection and dosing, and help you navigate potential interactions with conventional treatments.

3. Build a Supportive Network: Connect with other cancer patients, survivors, and caregivers who have experience with herbal medicine. Support groups, online forums, and community organizations can provide valuable insights, encouragement, and practical tips for incorporating herbal remedies into your cancer care routine.

4. Start Slowly and Gradually: Introduce herbal remedies into your routine gradually, starting with small doses and observing how your body responds. Keep a journal to track your symptoms, herb usage, and any changes in your health status over time. This can help you identify which herbs are most effective for your individual needs.

5. Focus on Whole Foods and Nutritional Support: Incorporate a variety of nutrient-rich whole foods into your diet, including fruits, vegetables, whole grains, legumes, nuts, seeds, and lean proteins. Herbal teas, smoothies, soups, and salads can be delicious ways to incorporate herbs into your meals and snacks.

6. Prioritize Stress Management and Self-Care: Explore relaxation techniques such as mindfulness meditation, deep breathing exercises, yoga, tai chi, and guided imagery to reduce stress, promote relaxation, and enhance emotional well-being. Herbal remedies such as adaptogens, nervines, and sedatives can also support stress resilience and promote restful sleep.

7. Support Digestive Health: Maintain digestive health by consuming a balanced diet, staying hydrated, and incorporating herbs that support digestion, such as ginger, peppermint, chamomile, fennel, and licorice. Probiotic-rich foods and supplements can also promote gut health and immune function.

8. Address Specific Symptoms and Side Effects: Identify specific symptoms and side effects you may be experiencing during cancer treatment, such as nausea, fatigue, pain, insomnia, or immune suppression. Work with your healthcare provider to select appropriate herbs and formulations to address these concerns.

9. Stay Informed and Stay Safe: Stay informed about potential herb-drug interactions, contraindications, and safety considerations. Inform your healthcare providers about any herbal remedies you are using to ensure they are compatible with your treatment plan and medical history.

10. Advocate for Yourself: Be proactive in advocating for your health and well-being. Ask questions, seek second opinions, and actively participate in decision-making about your care. Your healthcare team should respect your values, preferences, and treatment goals.

In conclusion, empowering yourself through herbal medicine involves taking an active role in your health and well-being, seeking support from qualified professionals, and incorporating practical strategies into your cancer care routine. By educating yourself, building a supportive network, focusing on nutrition and self-care, addressing specific symptoms, and staying informed and safe, you can harness the healing power of herbs to complement conventional cancer treatments and enhance your quality of life.

Lymphalin:

Definition: Lymphalin is a herbal supplement formulated to support lymphatic system health. The lymphatic system plays a crucial role in immune function and waste removal in the body, and Lymphalin is designed to promote its proper function.

Ingredients: Lymphalin typically contains a blend of herbs and botanical extracts known for their traditional use in supporting lymphatic system health. Common ingredients may include cleavers, red clover, echinacea, burdock root, and calendula, among others.

How to Prepare: Lymphalin is usually available in capsule or liquid form. Capsules are taken orally with water, while liquid forms may be mixed with water or juice before consumption. It's important to follow the recommended dosage on the product label.

Dosage: The appropriate dosage of Lymphalin can vary depending on the specific product and individual needs. It's important to follow the recommended dosage on the product label or consult with a healthcare professional for personalized guidance.

How to Use: Lymphalin capsules are typically taken orally with water, while liquid forms may be mixed with water or juice before consumption. It's often recommended to take Lymphalin on an empty stomach for optimal absorption.

Side Effects: Lymphalin is generally considered safe for most people when used as directed. However, some individuals may experience mild side effects such as gastrointestinal discomfort or allergic reactions to certain ingredients. It's important to consult with a healthcare provider before starting any new supplement regimen, especially if you have underlying health conditions or are taking medications.

Manjakani:

Definition: Manjakani, also known as Quercus infectoria or oak gall, is a natural substance derived from the oak tree. It has been used for centuries in traditional medicine for its potential health benefits, particularly for women's health and vaginal tightening.

Ingredients: Manjakani contains various bioactive compounds, including tannins, flavonoids, and gallic acid. These compounds are believed to contribute to the herb's medicinal properties, including its potential as an astringent and antiseptic agent.

How to Prepare: Manjakani is typically available in powder, capsule, or liquid extract form. It can be taken orally or used topically depending on the intended use. For vaginal tightening, manjakani may be applied topically as a gel or inserted into the vagina in capsule form.

Dosage: The appropriate dosage of manjakani can vary depending on factors such as age, health status, and the specific preparation being used. It's important to follow the recommended dosage on the product label or consult with a qualified herbalist or healthcare professional for personalized guidance.

How to Use: Manjakani can be taken orally or used topically depending on the intended use. It's important to use manjakani products as directed and to discontinue use if any adverse effects occur.

Side Effects: Manjakani is generally considered safe for most people when used in moderate amounts. However, some individuals may experience allergic reactions or skin irritation when used topically. It's important to use manjakani under the guidance of a healthcare professional and to discontinue use if any adverse effects occur.

Red Clover:

Definition: Red clover, scientifically known as Trifolium pratense, is a flowering plant belonging to the legume family. It's native to Europe, Western Asia, and Northwest Africa but has been naturalized in many other regions. Red clover has been used in traditional medicine for various purposes, including its potential to support women's health and menopausal symptoms.

Ingredients: Red clover contains several bioactive compounds, including isoflavones (such as genistein and daidzein), flavonoids, and phytoestrogens. These compounds are believed to contribute to the herb's medicinal properties, including its potential as a hormone-balancing agent and its ability to support cardiovascular health.

How to Prepare: Red clover is typically prepared and consumed as an herbal tea or tincture. To make tea, dried red clover flowers are steeped in hot water for several minutes before being strained and consumed. Tinctures are prepared by steeping the flowers in alcohol or vinegar to extract their active compounds.

Dosage: The appropriate dosage of red clover can vary depending on factors such as age, health status, and the specific preparation being used. It's important to follow the recommended dosage on the product label or consult with a qualified herbalist or healthcare professional for personalized guidance.

How to Use: Red clover tea or tincture is typically taken orally. It's important to use red clover products as directed and to discontinue use if any adverse effects occur.

Side Effects: Red clover is generally considered safe for most people when used in moderate amounts. However, some individuals may experience allergic reactions or digestive upset. It may also interact with certain medications or have adverse effects in individuals with certain health conditions. It's important to use red clover under the guidance of a healthcare professional and to discontinue use if any adverse effects occur.

Red Raspberry:

Definition: Red raspberry, scientifically known as Rubus idaeus, is a species of raspberry native to Europe and northern Asia. It's widely cultivated for its delicious berries and has been used in traditional medicine for various purposes, including its potential to support women's health during pregnancy and childbirth.

Ingredients: Red raspberry contains several bioactive compounds, including flavonoids, ellagic acid, anthocyanins, and vitamin C. These compounds are believed to contribute to the herb's medicinal properties, including its potential as an antioxidant, anti-inflammatory, and uterine tonic.

How to Prepare: Red raspberry leaf is typically prepared and consumed as an herbal tea or infusion. To make tea, dried red raspberry leaves are steeped in hot water for several minutes before being strained and consumed.

Dosage: The appropriate dosage of red raspberry leaf can vary depending on factors such as age, health status, and the specific preparation being used. It's important to follow the recommended dosage on the product label or consult with a qualified herbalist or healthcare professional for personalized guidance.

How to Use: Red raspberry leaf tea is typically taken orally. It's often recommended for pregnant individuals in the later stages of pregnancy to support uterine health and prepare for childbirth. It's important to use red raspberry leaf products as directed and to discontinue use if any adverse effects occur.

Side Effects: Red raspberry leaf is generally considered safe for most people when used in moderate amounts. However, some individuals may experience allergic reactions or digestive upset. Pregnant individuals should consult with a healthcare professional before using red raspberry leaf, especially if they have any underlying health conditions or are taking medications. It's important to use red raspberry leaf under the guidance of a healthcare professional and to discontinue use if any adverse effects occur.

Rhubarb:

Definition: Rhubarb, scientifically known as Rheum rhabarbarum, is a perennial plant cultivated for its edible stalks. While primarily used in culinary applications, rhubarb has also been utilized in traditional medicine for its potential health benefits, particularly for digestive health.

Ingredients: Rhubarb stalks contain various bioactive compounds, including anthraquinones (such as emodin and rhein), fiber, vitamins (such as vitamin K), and minerals (including calcium and potassium). These compounds are believed to contribute to the herb's medicinal properties, including its potential as a laxative and digestive aid.

How to Prepare: Rhubarb stalks are typically cooked before consumption, as the raw stalks are very tart and can be unpleasant to eat. They are often used in pies, crisps, jams, sauces, and other desserts, as well as in savory dishes. Rhubarb can also be used to make compotes, jams, and preserves.

Dosage: There is no specific dosage for rhubarb in culinary applications, as it is used as a food rather than a medicinal herb. However, when used for its potential laxative effects, it's important to consume rhubarb in moderation to avoid gastrointestinal upset.

How to Use: Rhubarb stalks can be chopped and cooked in various dishes, including pies, sauces, and jams. It's important to remove and discard the leaves, as they contain toxic compounds. When using rhubarb for its potential laxative effects, it's typically consumed as part of a cooked dish or in the form of a rhubarb-based herbal remedy.

Side Effects: Rhubarb stalks are generally safe for most people when consumed in moderate amounts as part of a balanced diet. However, excessive intake may lead to digestive upset or adverse effects due to the presence of oxalic acid, which can bind to calcium and form kidney stones in susceptible individuals. It's important to use rhubarb in moderation and to consult with a healthcare professional if you have any concerns or underlying health conditions.

Sarsaparilla:

Definition: Sarsaparilla refers to several species of plants belonging to the Smilax genus, including Smilax regelii and Smilax officinalis. It has been used historically in traditional medicine for its potential health benefits, particularly for its purported detoxifying and anti-inflammatory properties.

Ingredients: Sarsaparilla contains various bioactive compounds, including saponins (such as sarsaponin and smilagenin), flavonoids, phenolic acids, and sterols. These compounds are believed to contribute to the herb's medicinal properties, including its potential as a diuretic, blood purifier, and anti-inflammatory agent.

How to Prepare: Sarsaparilla root is typically prepared and consumed as an herbal tea, decoction, or tincture. To make tea, dried sarsaparilla root is steeped in hot water for several minutes before being strained and consumed. Decoctions involve boiling the root in water to extract its active compounds, while tinctures are prepared by steeping the root in alcohol or vinegar.

Dosage: The appropriate dosage of sarsaparilla can vary depending on factors such as age, health status, and the specific preparation being used. It's important to follow the recommended dosage on the product label or consult with a qualified herbalist or healthcare professional for personalized guidance.

How to Use: Sarsaparilla tea or tincture is typically taken orally. It's important to use sarsaparilla products as directed and to discontinue use if any adverse effects occur.

Side Effects: Sarsaparilla is generally considered safe for most people when used in moderate amounts. However, some individuals may experience allergic reactions or digestive upset. It may also interact with certain medications or have adverse effects in individuals with certain health conditions. It's important to use sarsaparilla under the guidance of a healthcare professional and to discontinue use if any adverse effects occur.

Tila:

Definition: Tila, also known as linden flower or lime blossom, refers to the flowers of the Tilia genus, primarily Tilia europaea and Tilia cordata. These trees are native to Europe, but they are also cultivated in other regions for their fragrant and medicinal flowers.

Ingredients: Tila flowers contain various bioactive compounds, including flavonoids, phenolic acids, and volatile oils. These compounds are believed to contribute to the herb's medicinal properties, including its potential as a mild sedative, anxiolytic, and anti-inflammatory agent.

How to Prepare: Tila flowers are typically prepared and consumed as an herbal tea or infusion. To make tea, dried tila flowers are steeped in hot water for several minutes before being strained and consumed.

Dosage: The appropriate dosage of tila can vary depending on factors such as age, health status, and the specific preparation being used. It's important to follow the recommended dosage on the product label or consult with a qualified herbalist or healthcare professional for personalized guidance.

How to Use: Tila tea is typically taken orally. It's often consumed in the evening as a calming bedtime beverage or during times of stress or anxiety. It's important to use tila products as directed and to discontinue use if any adverse effects occur.

Side Effects: Tila is generally considered safe for most people when used in moderate amounts. However, some individuals may experience allergic reactions or digestive upset. It may also interact with certain medications or have adverse effects in individuals with certain health conditions. It's important to use tila under the guidance of a healthcare professional and to discontinue use if any adverse effects occur.

Valerian:

Definition: Valerian, scientifically known as Valeriana officinalis, is a perennial flowering plant native to Europe and Asia. It has been used for centuries in traditional medicine for its potential calming and sedative effects.

Ingredients: Valerian root contains several bioactive compounds, including valerenic acid, valepotriates, and volatile oils. These compounds are believed to contribute to the herb's medicinal properties, including its potential as a sedative, anxiolytic, and sleep aid.

How to Prepare: Valerian root is typically prepared and consumed as an herbal tea, tincture, or capsule. To make tea, dried valerian root is steeped in hot water for several minutes before being strained and consumed. Tinctures are prepared by steeping the root in alcohol or vinegar to extract its active compounds.

Dosage: The appropriate dosage of valerian can vary depending on factors such as age, health status, and the specific preparation being used. It's important to follow the recommended dosage on the product label or consult with a qualified herbalist or healthcare professional for personalized guidance.

How to Use: Valerian tea, tincture, or capsules are typically taken orally. It's often consumed in the evening as a sleep aid or during times of stress or anxiety. It's important to use valerian products as directed and to discontinue use if any adverse effects occur.

Side Effects: Valerian is generally considered safe for most people when used in moderate amounts. However, some individuals may experience mild side effects such as drowsiness, headache, or gastrointestinal upset. It may also interact with certain medications or have adverse effects in individuals with certain health conditions. It's important to use valerian under the guidance of a healthcare professional and to discontinue use if any adverse effects occur.

Wild Cherry Bark:

Definition: Wild cherry bark, scientifically known as Prunus serotina, is the bark obtained from the black cherry tree native to North America. It has been used traditionally in Native American and folk medicine for its potential health benefits, particularly for respiratory and digestive issues.

Ingredients: Wild cherry bark contains various bioactive compounds, including cyanogenic glycosides (such as prunasin and amygdalin), flavonoids, and phenolic acids. These compounds are believed to contribute to the herb's medicinal properties, including its potential as an expectorant, cough suppressant, and mild sedative.

How to Prepare: Wild cherry bark is typically prepared and consumed as an herbal tea, decoction, or syrup. To make tea, dried wild cherry bark is steeped in hot water for several minutes before being strained and consumed. Decoctions involve boiling the bark in water to extract its active compounds, while syrups are made by simmering the bark with sugar or honey to create a thick, sweet liquid.

Dosage: The appropriate dosage of wild cherry bark can vary depending on factors such as age, health status, and the specific preparation being used. It's important to follow the recommended dosage on the product label or consult with a qualified herbalist or healthcare professional for personalized guidance.

How to Use: Wild cherry bark tea, decoction, or syrup is typically taken orally. It's often consumed to soothe coughs, sore throats, and other respiratory symptoms. It's important to use wild cherry bark products as directed and to discontinue use if any adverse effects occur.

Side Effects: Wild cherry bark is generally considered safe for most people when used in moderate amounts. However, it contains cyanogenic glycosides, which can release cyanide in the body when metabolized. While the risk of cyanide poisoning from consuming wild cherry bark is low when used appropriately, excessive intake or prolonged use may lead to adverse effects. It's important to use wild cherry bark under the guidance of a healthcare professional and to discontinue use if any adverse effects occur.

Yellowdock:

Definition: Yellowdock, scientifically known as Rumex crispus, is a perennial flowering plant native to Europe and western Asia but is also found in North America. It has a long history of use in traditional medicine, particularly among Indigenous peoples, for its potential health benefits.

Ingredients: Yellowdock root contains various bioactive compounds, including anthraquinone glycosides (such as emodin and chrysophanol), tannins, and vitamins (including vitamin A and vitamin C). These compounds are believed to contribute to the herb's medicinal properties, including its potential as a laxative, blood cleanser, and liver tonic.

How to Prepare: Yellowdock root is typically prepared and consumed as an herbal tea, tincture, or capsule. To make tea, dried yellowdock root is steeped in hot water for several minutes before being strained and consumed. Tinctures are prepared by steeping the root in alcohol or vinegar to extract its active compounds.

Dosage: The appropriate dosage of yellowdock can vary depending on factors such as age, health status, and the specific preparation being used. It's important to follow the recommended dosage on the product label or consult with a qualified herbalist or healthcare professional for personalized guidance.

How to Use: Yellowdock tea, tincture, or capsules are typically taken orally. It's often consumed to support digestion, promote bowel regularity, and cleanse the blood. It's important to use yellowdock products as directed and to discontinue use if any adverse effects occur.

Side Effects: Yellowdock is generally considered safe for most people when used in moderate amounts. However, some individuals may experience mild side effects such as gastrointestinal upset or allergic reactions. It may also interact with certain medications or have adverse effects in individuals with certain health conditions. It's important to use yellowdock under the guidance of a healthcare professional and to discontinue use if any adverse effects occur.

Yellowdock Root:

Definition: Yellowdock root, scientifically known as Rumex crispus, is the root of a perennial flowering plant native to Europe and western Asia, also found in North America. It has a long history of use in traditional medicine, particularly among Indigenous peoples, for its potential health benefits.

Ingredients: Yellowdock root contains various bioactive compounds, including anthraquinone glycosides (such as emodin and chrysophanol), tannins, and vitamins (including vitamin A and vitamin C). These compounds are believed to contribute to the herb's medicinal properties, including its potential as a laxative, blood cleanser, and liver tonic.

How to Prepare: Yellowdock root is typically prepared and consumed as an herbal tea, tincture, or capsule. To make tea, dried yellowdock root is steeped in hot water for several minutes before being strained and consumed. Tinctures are prepared by steeping the root in alcohol or vinegar to extract its active compounds.

Dosage: The appropriate dosage of yellowdock root can vary depending on factors such as age, health status, and the specific preparation being used. It's important to follow the recommended dosage on the product label or consult with a qualified herbalist or healthcare professional for personalized guidance.

How to Use: Yellowdock root tea, tincture, or capsules are typically taken orally. It's often consumed to support digestion, promote bowel regularity, and cleanse the blood. It's important to use yellowdock root products as directed and to discontinue use if any adverse effects occur.

Side Effects: Yellowdock root is generally considered safe for most people when used in moderate amounts. However, some individuals may experience mild side effects such as gastrointestinal upset or allergic reactions. It may also interact with certain medications or have adverse effects in individuals with certain health conditions. It's important to use yellowdock root under the guidance of a healthcare professional and to discontinue use if any adverse effects occur.

Agrimony:

Definition: Agrimony, scientifically known as Agrimonia eupatoria, is a perennial herbaceous plant native to Europe, Asia, and North America. It has a long history of use in traditional medicine, particularly in European folk medicine, for its potential health benefits.

Ingredients: Agrimony contains various bioactive compounds, including tannins, flavonoids, phenolic acids, and volatile oils. These compounds are believed to contribute to the herb's medicinal properties, including its potential as an astringent, anti-inflammatory, and digestive aid.

How to Prepare: Agrimony is typically prepared and consumed as an herbal tea, tincture, or poultice. To make tea, dried agrimony leaves and flowers are steeped in hot water for several minutes before being strained and consumed. Tinctures are prepared by steeping the herb in alcohol or vinegar to extract its active compounds.

Dosage: The appropriate dosage of agrimony can vary depending on factors such as age, health status, and the specific preparation being used. It's important to follow the recommended dosage on the product label or consult with a qualified herbalist or healthcare professional for personalized guidance.

How to Use: Agrimony tea, tincture, or poultice is typically taken orally or applied topically. It's often consumed to soothe gastrointestinal issues, such as indigestion and diarrhea, or used externally to treat skin conditions.

Side Effects: Agrimony is generally considered safe for most people when used in moderate amounts. However, some individuals may experience allergic reactions or gastrointestinal upset. It may also interact with certain medications or have adverse effects in individuals with certain health conditions. It's important to use agrimony under the guidance of a healthcare professional and to discontinue use if any adverse effects occur.

Alfalfa:

Definition: Alfalfa, scientifically known as Medicago sativa, is a flowering plant in the pea family native to Asia but cultivated worldwide. It's primarily grown as fodder for livestock, but it has also been used in traditional medicine for its potential health benefits.

Ingredients: Alfalfa contains various bioactive compounds, including vitamins (such as vitamin A, vitamin C, and vitamin K), minerals (including calcium, magnesium, and potassium), amino acids, and phytoestrogens. These compounds are believed to contribute to the herb's medicinal properties, including its potential as a nutritive tonic, diuretic, and hormone balancer.

How to Prepare: Alfalfa is typically consumed as sprouts, herbal tea, or in supplement form (such as capsules or tablets). To make tea, dried alfalfa leaves are steeped in hot water for several minutes before being strained and consumed.

Dosage: The appropriate dosage of alfalfa can vary depending on factors such as age, health status, and the specific preparation being used. It's important to follow the recommended dosage on the product label or consult with a qualified herbalist or healthcare professional for personalized guidance.

How to Use: Alfalfa sprouts, tea, or supplements are typically taken orally. It's often consumed as a dietary supplement to support overall health and well-being, as well as to promote kidney health and hormone balance.

Side Effects: Alfalfa is generally considered safe for most people when consumed in moderate amounts. However, some individuals may experience allergic reactions or digestive upset. It may also interact with certain medications or have adverse effects in individuals with certain health conditions, such as autoimmune diseases or hormone-sensitive conditions. Pregnant or breastfeeding individuals should consult with a healthcare professional before using alfalfa supplements. It's important to use alfalfa under the guidance of a healthcare professional and to discontinue use if any adverse effects occur.

Ashwagandha:

Definition: Ashwagandha, scientifically known as Withaniasomnifera, is a small shrub native to India, the Middle East, and parts of Africa. It has a long history of use in Ayurvedic medicine for its potential health benefits, particularly for its adaptogenic properties.

Ingredients: Ashwagandha root contains various bioactive compounds, including alkaloids (such as withanolides), steroidal lactones, and flavonoids. These compounds are believed to contribute to the herb's medicinal properties, including its potential as an adaptogen, anti-inflammatory, and immune-modulating agent.

How to Prepare: Ashwagandha is typically consumed as a powdered root, herbal tea, tincture, or in supplement form (such as capsules or tablets). To make tea, dried ashwagandha root is steeped in hot water for several minutes before being strained and consumed.

Dosage: The appropriate dosage of ashwagandha can vary depending on factors such as age, health status, and the specific preparation being used. It's important to follow the recommended dosage on the product label or consult with a qualified herbalist or healthcare professional for personalized guidance.

How to Use: Ashwagandha powder, tea, tincture, or supplements are typically taken orally. It's often consumed to support stress management, promote relaxation, and boost overall vitality and well-being.

Side Effects: Ashwagandha is generally considered safe for most people when used in moderate amounts. However, some individuals may experience mild side effects such as gastrointestinal upset or drowsiness. It may also interact with certain medications or have adverse effects in individuals with certain health conditions, such as autoimmune diseases or thyroid disorders. Pregnant or breastfeeding individuals should consult with a healthcare professional before using ashwagandha supplements. It's important to use ashwagandha under the guidance of a healthcare professional and to discontinue use if any adverse effects occur.

Astragalus:

Definition: Astragalus, scientifically known as Astragalus membranaceus, is a flowering plant native to China and Mongolia but also found in other parts of Asia. It has been used for centuries in traditional Chinese medicine for its potential health benefits, particularly for its immune-enhancing properties.

Ingredients: Astragalus root contains various bioactive compounds, including polysaccharides, saponins (such as astragalosides), flavonoids, and amino acids. These compounds are believed to contribute to the herb's medicinal properties, including its potential as an adaptogen, immunomodulator, and anti-inflammatory agent.

How to Prepare: Astragalus is typically consumed as a powdered root, herbal tea, tincture, or in supplement form (such as capsules or tablets). To make tea, dried astragalus root slices are simmered in water for several minutes before being strained and consumed.

Dosage: The appropriate dosage of astragalus can vary depending on factors such as age, health status, and the specific preparation being used. It's important to follow the recommended dosage on the product label or consult with a qualified herbalist or healthcare professional for personalized guidance.

How to Use: Astragalus powder, tea, tincture, or supplements are typically taken orally. It's often consumed to support immune function, promote vitality, and enhance overall well-being.

Side Effects: Astragalus is generally considered safe for most people when used in moderate amounts. However, some individuals may experience mild side effects such as gastrointestinal upset or allergic reactions. It may also interact with certain medications or have adverse effects in individuals with certain health conditions, such as autoimmune diseases or diabetes. Pregnant or breastfeeding individuals should consult with a healthcare professional before using astragalus supplements. It's important to use astragalus under the guidance of a healthcare professional and to discontinue use if any adverse effects occur.

THE END

www.ingramcontent.com/pod-product-compliance
Lightning Source LLC
Chambersburg PA
CBHW081558250726
48653CB00009B/3481